S. MATHEWS

Essential Oils: Beginners Guide for Moms

Oils for Family Health & Wellness

First edition

This book was professionally typeset on Reedsy.
Find out more at reedsy.com

This book is dedicated to my husband and three children, who have been my support and champions. I especially want to thank my daughter, JMV, who has been my graphic designer and technical superstar. I love you all with all my heart.
I thank God for this amazing opportunity. It has been a great experience and I can't wait for the journey ahead.

Contents

One

Introduction

Welcome to the Essential Oils: Beginner's Guide for Moms; Essential Oils for Family Health and Wellness. This book is a comprehensive resource for using essential oils to promote family health and wellness. In this book, you can expect to learn about the many benefits of using essential oils, including how they can support physical and emotional health. I will cover the history of essential oils and how to use essential oils for different concerns, such as sleep, stress, body pain, and skin care. You will also learn about specific essential oils that are safe for children and tips on how to incorporate essential oils into your daily routine and self-care practices.

My goal is to provide you with the knowledge and resources you need to use essential oils safely and effectively for a happier and healthier life. This book is only a small version of essential oils' benefits for your family. It is a quick guide you can reference in those 'oh no" moments when your child may have a runny nose, trouble sleeping or other minor health issues. This book is also a valuable resource for mothers looking to practice self-care and support their wellness, and wind down, especially after long and tiring days. This guide also includes some brief information on oils to use for the men in our lives. It also explores the ways to use essential oils and using essential oils for a chemical-free environment. There is also an essential oil glossary with a list of oils from A-Z for you to check out.

Essential oils are derived from plants and have a wide range of benefits, from boosting immunity to promoting relaxation and improving mood. Essential oils are different from other oils in many different ways. They are oils extracted from plants by steam distillation, cold pressing, and solvent extraction. There are many types of oils produced by pressing the seeds of the nuts of plants. Essential oils have high concentration levels and are highly potent and are commonly used in aromatherapy, natural medical treatments, and personal care products.

While essential oils have many benefits, they can also have potential risks and side effects when misused. Healthcare professionals should be consulted before use and for any questions, especially when using it on children.

As a mother of three children, I know how important it is to keep children happy and healthy. However, I only found natural and effective ways to do so once I discovered the power of essential oils. I have experienced the many benefits of essential oils in my family's daily routines. My essential oil journey started in 2012 when my daughter was born, and I gradually started using light and safe oils on myself as a first-time mother. I noticed the small benefits in my immunity when I felt under the weather. I later started to use baby-safe oils on my daughter when she was a toddler when I felt she needed an immunity boost or to help when she was sick. Over time, I became more comfortable and confident using essential oils and discovered their incredible potential for supporting family health. I use essential oils for my family to give me peace of mind that I'm using natural ways to heal and support my family's health and wellness.

Imagine using all-natural products to help all those minor health issues in those cold winter seasons. Essential oils can be the go-to product you can grab from the cabinet and help your family members have that extra protection and peace of mind to have your loved ones feeling well.

Now in 2023, I continue to use essential oils on all my three children, my husband, and myself. I use essential oils in my daily routine and life, from morning drops of lemon oil in my water to applying lavender oil on the kids at bedtime for good sleep. I hope you find this a helpful guide and use it in your family life as I have done with mine and see all the incredible benefits it shows in your journey towards wellness.

I'm excited to write this book because I want to share the many benefits I have seen in using essential oils and to be able to share this knowledge with others. My personal experiences and passion for using essential oils to promote wellness in my family have motivated me to share my knowledge and insight with other mothers looking for safe and natural ways to enhance the health and well-being of their loved ones. I hope this guide provides helpful information and encourages readers to explore the many benefits of essential oils for family health and wellness. I hope you can take any part of this book and use it for yourself or anyone in your family and give a natural way to help your family stay healthy.

Two

History of Essential Oils: Overall Benefits on young children

Essential oils are a class of volatile oils that give plants their characteristic odors, which are used in perfumes and aromatherapy. [1] These oils have been used all through the world since ancient times. It is documented in various cultures, including ancient Egypt, India, Greece, and China. Essential oils have existed since ancient times, dating back to 2500 B.C. The old and new testaments in the Bible have many references to plants derived from essential oils, and many are used in the Bible. Many countries around the world have an early reference to using essential oils. Ancient Egyptians used essential oils often for medicinal benefits and also beauty. The famous Cleopatra is said to have used many essential oils. Greece is also a known country with a history of using essential oils. Hippocrats is a Greek physician known as the "Father of modern medicine." He studied plants' influence on medicine and applied it to his healing treatments. Some oils, such as frankincense essential oils, known as "the king of essential oils," are more valued than gold. [14]

In India, essential oils have been a central part of the Indian Ayurvedic health system. The principles of Ayurveda are a view of natural healing that incorporates the application of oils. China also uses many plants and herbs in their healing traditions, including acupuncture. [4]

There are many benefits to using essential oils. Essential oils have been applied to children to fight many health problems and support immunity. The changing weather in the seasons makes children more susceptible to catching viruses. Specific essential oils can help target particular symptoms making children feel better during those cold seasons. Parents can use essential oils to help their children in the areas to improve sleep, for stomach or body pain, manage moods and emotions, and so much more.

Three

Safety Precaution of oils/ Use of essential oils for young children/ Carrier oils

There are many essential oils to promote wellness. It is very important to be careful and research the essential oil you want to use on children. Many oils can be classified as "hot," and diluting them with a carrier oil will balance things and make them more tolerable and effective. Hot oils illustrate as having a burning or uncomfortable feeling on the skin or eyes, which indicates that the oil is too strong and needs dilution of carrier oil. You should not apply essential oils without precaution, and always consult a medical provider to ensure it is safe. There are essential oil safety guidelines that are reviewed when using essential oils on children. Here are some safety guidelines to keep in mind when using essential oils on children:

Always dilute the essential oil with a carrier oil before applying it on a child's skin. The recommended dilution ratio is 1-2 drops of essential oil per 1 tablespoon of carrier oil.[8] Carrier oils can help dilute the essential oil so it is not as strong and makes it more tolerable for children. Here are a few common carrier oils that can be used with essential oils when diluting for children.

- Fractionated coconut oil
- Sweet almond oil
- Jojoba oil

Several essential oils are not recommended for use on children. Along with the great oils to apply on children, there are also some oils to avoid on younger children. Following safety guidelines and using carrier oils to dilute potent oils can help you use essential oils safely and effectively to promote wellness for your children and family.

- Peppermint oil: It can be too intense for children, especially those under age 6. It can cause skin irritation, respiratory distress, and even seizures are possible.

- Wintergreen oil contains a high concentration of methyl salicylate, which can cause respiratory distress.

- Oregano oil is a potent essential oil that has several health benefits. It is powerful and can cause skin irritation or allergic reactions in children. Children with asthma or respiratory problems should avoid oregano oil as it can cause respiratory distress. It's important to always dilute oregano oil with a carrier oil and use it in small amounts on children.

- Tea tree oil is a popular oil and has many benefits. It is a strong oil that should be diluted on children due to skin irritation. Children should only use tea tree oils in small amounts.

When using essential oils, it is important to follow specific guidelines to ensure their safe and effective use. You should understand the importance of proper dilution ratios and application. It is also important to know of any potential safety risks or side effects associated with specific oils. Some oils can cause skin sensitivity or allergic reactions in some individuals.

Your healthcare provider can give guidance and advice on the safe and appropriate use of essential oils for your individual needs. You should consult a health care provider before using essential oils, especially if you are pregnant, nursing, or have a pre-existing medical condition. By adhering to safety procedures and understanding essential oils' potential risks and benefits, you can safely and effectively use these powerful natural remedies to enhance your health and well-being.

There is research on the health benefits of essential oils. The FDA doesn't monitor or regulate essential oils, so it's important to talk with a healthcare provider before using them and discuss how you plan on using them. A few factors to look at when using essential oils are age, health conditions, and method of using oils.

Four

Top essential oils that are safe for children

Moms look for the best ways to take care of their family members and children are a top priority. It is a great tool to have a list of the top essential oils to grab and use in those times to keep children healthy. Being safe and following precautions on using essential oils is especially important when using on young children. Essential oils are recommended for ages two and above, although there are safe oils that can be used for infants.

Below are some of the top oils that are gentle for children who are two and above. There are a variety of gentler oils that are safe for newborns to age two years. When using essential oils, it is very important to dilute them with a carrier oil because many oils have a strong potency, making them harder to handle on children. If the oil is too strong, it can tingle or make the eyes watery or sting. A carrier oil balance will help make the essential oil feel gentle when applied to avoid those effects. Here are a few significant "go-to" oils for children.

Lavender Essential Oil has anti-inflammatory, antifungal, antidepressant, antibacterial, and antimicrobial properties. It's a very gentle oil, especially for children, to help with many daily things

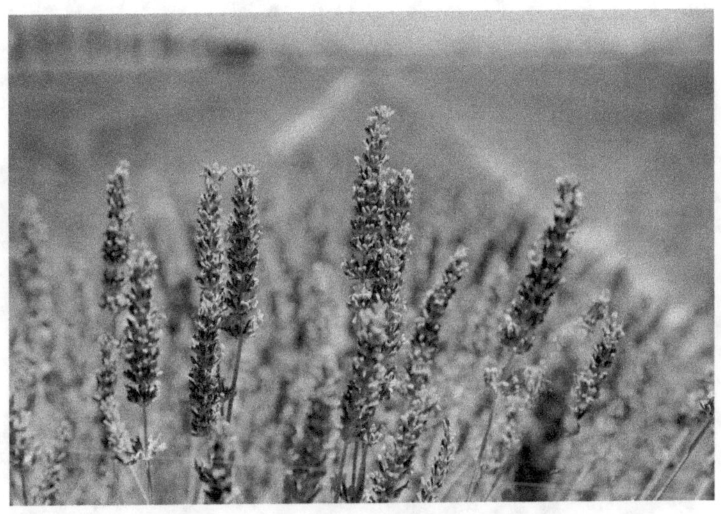

- **Uses**: to help kids have a good night's sleep, helps reduce anxiety levels; used for cuts, bruises, and burns; seasonal respiratory health
- **Scent**: floral, sweet, fresh

Frankincense Essential Oil is an aromatic resin used in many perfumes and incense. Dilution is recommended for children that use frankincense oil.

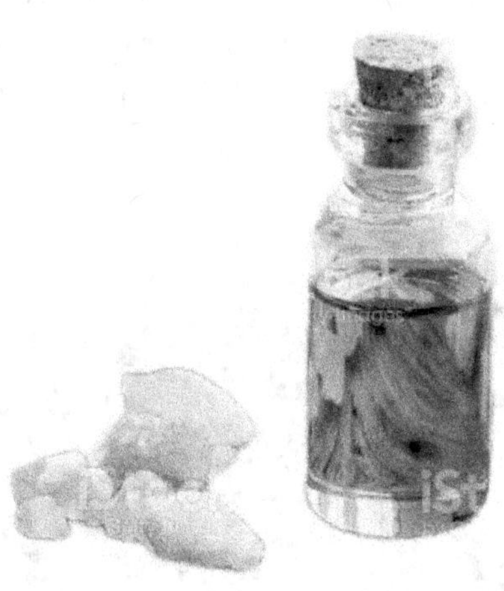

Uses: immune support, soothes coughs, and respiratory infections

Scent: the combination of pine and lemon, woodsy

Roman Chamomile Oil has antibacterial and antimicrobial properties. It's a gentle oil that calms and soothes children.

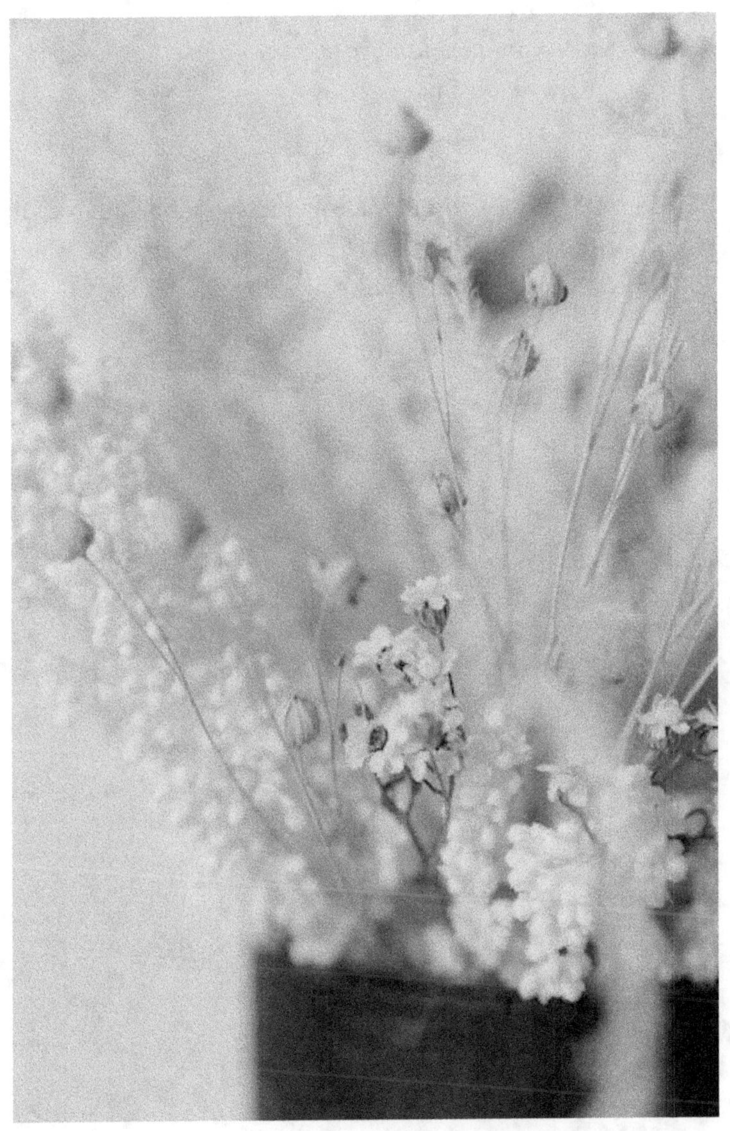

Uses: treats common cold, sore throat
Scent: apple-like aroma

Lemon Oil is a safe oil for children and should be diluted. It can be sensitive to direct sunlight and cause skin irritation, and you should be appropriately diluted with a carrier oil.

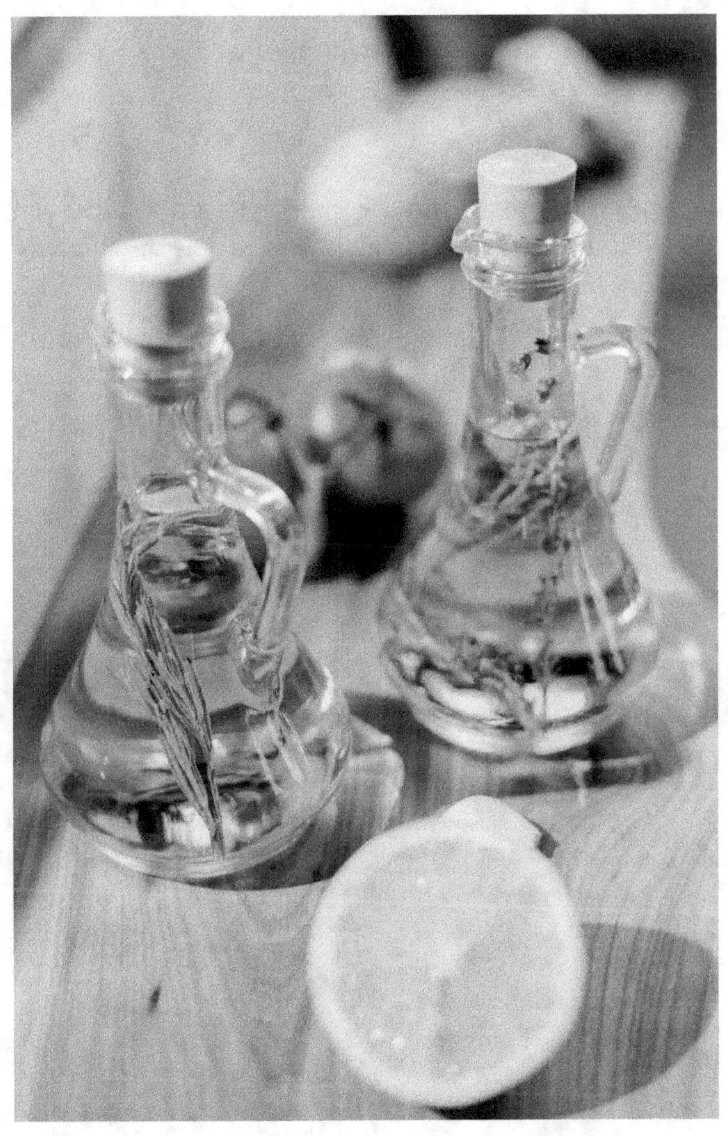

Uses: improve cold symptoms, helps sore throats
Scent: fresh lemons

Eucalyptus Oil comes from the leaves of the Eucalyptus plant and is an antiseptic used in ointments and other products for healing.

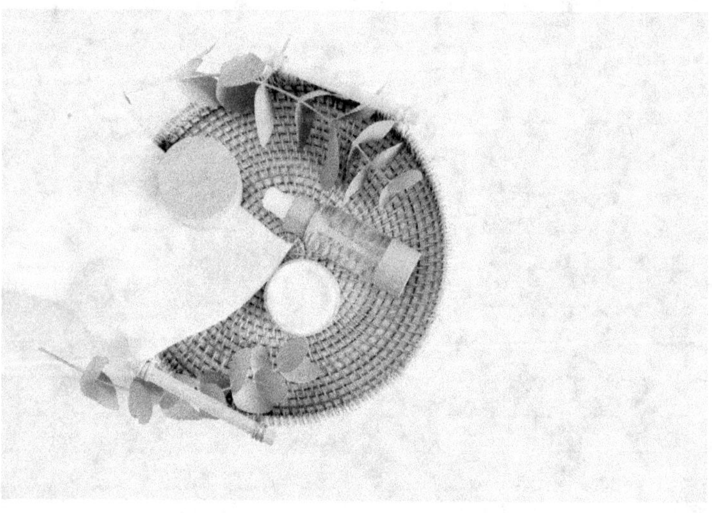

Uses: cough reliever, muscle and joint pain
Scent: minty, citrus, fresh, clean

It is great to have a toolbox of oils to reference when mothers need to know which oils can target specific health issues and areas to help with different struggles in life. Essential oils are an alternative to sometimes reaching for OTC (over-the-counter) medications and can aid in the following issues.

Essential oils for the common cold

The common cold and its symptoms in kids can cause added stress to any mom. It can mean kids miss school and also parents have to miss work. Some great essential oils to use when you see the starting signs of the sniffles and cold are:

Eucalyptus oil: it has decongestant properties that can help with a stuffy nose

Lavender oil: has calming properties that can help kids sleep better

Lemon oil: has antiviral properties that can boost the immune system

Essential oils for allergy season

Allergy season can be another area where essential oils can help with those symptoms which are triggered due to the change in season.

Peppermint oil: has anti-inflammatory properties that can assist with nasal congestion and sinus discomfort. It helps with headaches that can be associated with allergies.

Lemon oil: has antihistamine properties that can help relieve allergy symptoms such as itchy eyes and runny nose.

Essential oils for a better sleep [10]

Everyone can benefit from a good night's sleep. Sleep in your household is a very important need regardless of age. Children not getting enough sleep can affect their mood, physical health, and wellness. Sleep is also very important for moms to function and care for their families. Many oils can help children be calm and relaxed for a good night's sleep at the end of the day.

- Lavender oil
- Frankincense oil

Essential oils for cuts, wounds, and bruises

Along the road of life, children have their share of falls, scrapes, burns, and bruises. The mother is often the go-to person kids run to get those boo-boos taken care of and to make them all better. Some essential oils can help make those cuts, scrapes, and burns feel better and get your child back on their feet to play and enjoy the fun times ahead. [11]

- Lavender oil is versatile and helps heal many things, i.e., cuts, scrapes, burns, wounds, and scars. Lavender is a great go-to oil to put on a cut for healing. Applying a drop of lavender oil on a bandaid before covering a cut is also good to promote natural healing.
- Tea tree oil has the power to treat wounds as an antiseptic and helps with the cleaning aspect to help prevent infection.
- Frankincense oil has a variety of medicinal properties. It can help with cell and skin rejuvenation. Do not apply directly on an open cut; it is a potent oil.
- Lemon Oil is an oil used as a clearing agent with antibacterial properties. It's a good oil for disinfecting and cleaning wounds and is also an oil that needs dilution due to its strength.
- Peppermint Oil has analgesic properties, which can help

alleviate pain. It can also protect the scrape or wound from germs.

Essential oils for stomach aches

Several essential oils can help alleviate stomach aches and digestive discomfort. When using essential oils for stomach issues, it is important to dilute them properly. They can be applied topically to the stomach and added to a warm compress for relief. Below are a few oils to consider.

- Peppermint oil has been researched and used to help aid in stomach problems. It can help reduce nausea and bloating. It is a potent oil and should be diluted for children.
- Ginger oil can help ease digestive issues. It can reduce nausea, bloating, and gas.
- Chamomile oil has anti-inflammatory properties that can calm digestive inflammation. It can calm and reduce nausea and relax the stomach.
- Lemon oil can improve digestion and help alleviate nausea and bloating.
- Fennel oil can help relieve digestive discomfort and bloating. It can also stimulate digestion.

Five

Top Essential Oils for Mothers

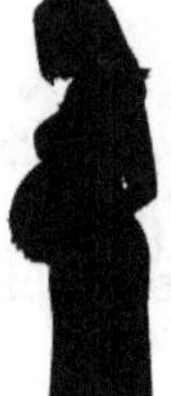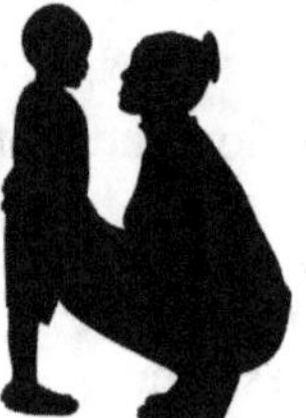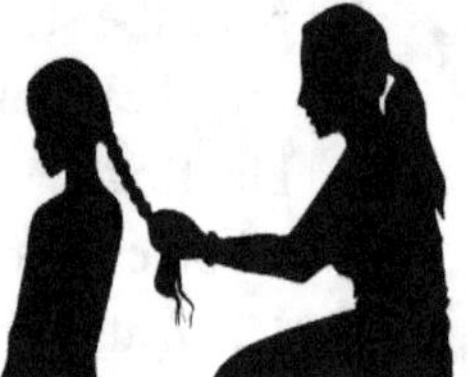

Essential oils can benefit all types of moms, from the pregnant mom to the grandma taking care of her grandchild. Precautions should be taken when using certain essential oils, especially during pregnancy and certain medications. It is a good idea to consult a medical provider and inform them if you are using essential oils and to get guidance on the safety measures.

Pregnant moms:

- Lavender oil: It is a gentle essential oil that can help calm and soothe the mind and body. It is an excellent choice for relieving stress, anxiety, and insomnia, which are common issues for pregnant women
- Frankincense oil: Promotes relaxation and relieves during pregnancy. It can support skin care, which can help prevent stretch marks.
- Chamomile oil: Gentle oil to soothe the mind and mood. It can relieve anxiety, insomnia, and digestive issues during pregnancy

Moms of infants/ toddlers:

- Lavender oil: Gentle and calming oil that can help relax moms and toddlers. It's a go-to choice for getting restful sleep, reducing stress, and relieving minor skin irritations
- Eucalyptus oil: Promotes respiratory health and clears congestion in toddlers. It also boosts energy and mental clarity for moms.
- Lemon oil: Boosts immune systems for mom and toddler. It's a safe oil choice for cleaning your home.
- Tea tree oil: Treats minor cuts, scrapes, and skin irritations in both moms and toddlers

Moms of teens:

- Lavender Oil: This oil has calming and relaxing properties that may help reduce stress and anxiety and to promote better sleep which is very important for moms and teenagers.
- Lemon Oil: This oil has uplifting and energizing properties that boost mood, improve focus and reduce stress.
- Ylang ylang: It can enhance moods and help reduce feelings of tension, and irritability, and promotes relaxation.

Grandmoms:

- Frankincense Oil: This oil has anti-inflammatory properties that can help with joint pain and arthritis, which can be concerning for many grandmoms
- Peppermint Oil: It can help with headaches, indigestion, and fatigue
- Rosemary Oil: has memory-enhancing properties and can help improve cognitive function and focus as women age.

Essential oils also benefit mothers seeking ways to care for themselves and practice self-care. It can help strengthen immunity, and pain management, boost mood, and provide emotional support. Mothers can also use many essential oils in their houses to offer non-toxic alternatives in daily laundry, washing dishes, and cleaning floors. There are many oils for the day-in and day-out of the busy lives of mothers. Taking care of your whole body and how you live your life is so important. Mothers tend to have the "care for my family before me" view.

Essential oils can be a natural addition to your home and can be used in small steps to make a big difference.

When caring for children and families, mothers should have a healthy immune system, and essential oils can aid in that a healthy mother is a happy mother who can be available to her family and stay in good health. Thieves, lemon, and Peppermint oils are a few good oils to assist in helping mothers' respiratory systems during the fall and winter months.

Another system of support is keeping a healthy weight and how mothers often have a hard time losing weight, especially after having children. A few oils that can help manage weight are Grapefruit essential oil, Peppermint, and Lemon. Vitality oils can be ingested and are a safe option for adding oil to water or food.

Along with your physical well-being, supporting your emotional well-being is also very important. Essential oils can help with many mothers' stressful and busy schedules daily. Moms need to have those relaxation moments after their busy mom moments. Oils that can help with emotional support include stress away, lemon, peppermint, and frankincense. Other oils that have helped with mood-enhancing include bergamot, patchouli, rose, sandalwood, ylang,ylang. These oils that can help enhance moods can give calming and uplifting effects.

Mood Moments :

1. A few drops of lavender oil can be added to a warm bath to relax.

2. Peppermint oil can be diffused in the morning to help with alertness and focus.
3. Applying essential oils to the wrist and temples can help during stressful times.

Skincare and promoting healthy aging can be a concern as mothers balance the many facets of work and home life. Beauty and health can often be forgotten, and stress appears on your face. After having children, life gets extra busy, and self-care for your skin is so important. Here are a few tips on how to use essential oils for skin support. [13]

- Tip 1: Frankincense essential oil is an excellent oil for all skin types. It has anti-inflammatory and antibacterial benefits that can help skin that is prone to acne or blemishes. It can be used as an astringent to decrease large pores and to even out skin tone. Use frankincense oil by adding a few drops to your body lotion and apply it wherever you feel a boost is needed.

-

- Tip 2: Rose essential oil is a wonder oil that has properties that reduce redness and puffiness in the skin. It is an oil known to be high in vitamins C and E. You can add rose oil to your facial products or apply it straight. It's a great source to keep your skin looking youthful and healthy.

-

- Tip 3: Ylang Ylang essential oil [12] - Ylang ylang essential oil is from a flower that is often in the top notes of perfumes. It can be used as a moisturizer for dry skin. You should use a skin test for this oil to see if it causes any irritation.

•

• Tip 4: Lavender essential oil is a versatile oil that is used for many things. For moms, lavender can be added to creams for skin care in the areas of unclogging pores, healing acne, and reducing any inflammation. It is a gentle oil and can be applied directly to spots on the face. As oils react differently for every person, it's important to do a skin test to see if there is any reaction. Adding a few drops of lavender oil to a warm bath can help relax moms and soak away the day's stress. The minimal stress can then lead to a better night's sleep.

A big support system that can oftentimes be forgotten is the importance of having healthy sleep habits. Mothers can constantly overload their thoughts and keep their minds busy, even when it's time to turn them off and go to bed. Oils that are great to help with sleep include; lavender, ylang ylang, vetiver, roman chamomile, and frankincense. These oils have the option of being diffused or applied topically

Essential oils for men

Many different types of people can use essential oils. Men may have a different view on using essential oils, but the benefits of using essential oils for men can be just as wonderful. We can't forget about the men in our lives, along with the mothers and children. Essential oils can benefit men in various ways, such as promoting relaxation and boosting energy levels. Here are a few oils for men to feel well the natural way. [9]

- Vetiver is an oil that is used in many colognes. It has an earthy, spicy smell which can be great for calming stress and anxiety.

- Copaiba is another oil that men can apply. It has a warm smell that can be applied before bedtime on the feet to get relaxed before bedtime. Copaiba is also used to boost skin health.

- Tea tree oil is an excellent oil to combat odors for socks and shoes. It has properties to be anti-fungal and take away bad smells.

- Cedarwood oil is a warm, grounding oil that boosts confidence and self-esteem. It's a great oil to use before exercising and working out. It also helps soothe sore muscles after a workout. It also has a warm and comforting scent that can improve sleep, balance emotions, and improve concentration.

- Frankincense oil has a rich and grounding aroma that can promote relaxation and reduce stress. It can support the immune system and help keep the skin healthy.

- Black pepper essential oil has a spicy scent that can increase energy levels and improve circulation. It can help reduce muscle and joint pain.

Seven

Ways to use essential oils

There are three main ways of using essential oils:

1. Applying them topically
2. Diffusing them in a diffuser
3. Inhaling them directly or using aromatherapy jewelry

Using essential oils can be a great way to enjoy their therapeutic benefits. It's important to use essential oils safely and know their strengths. Here are some tips on how to use essential oils safely and effectively.

Topical Application:

One way to use oils is by applying them topically to the skin. You can apply oils easily with a rollerball to avoid making a mess. Before applying an essential oil topically, it's wise to check for sensitivity or allergic reactions by diluting the oils with a skin patch test on your inner arm before applying the oil to a larger area of your skin. Wait 24-48 hours to see if there is any sensitivity before applying it to a larger skin area. Dilute the oil with a carrier oil to reduce its strength and minimize the risk of skin irritation.

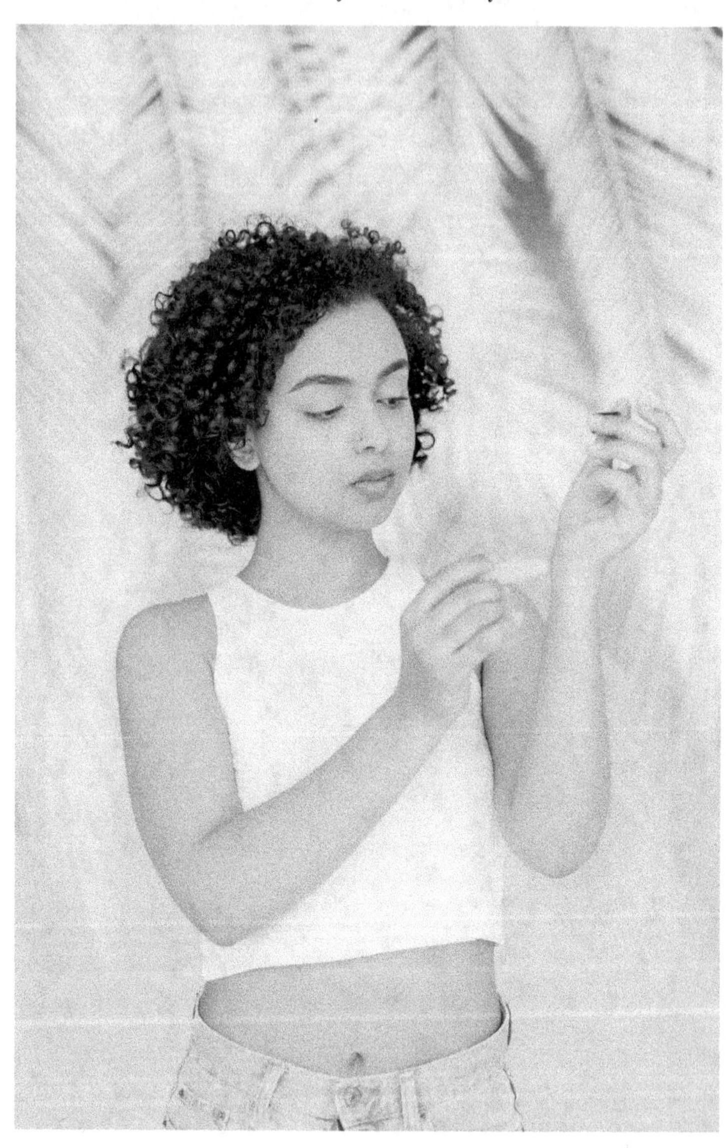

Diffusion:

Another way to use essential oils is by diffusing the oils in a diffuser. A diffuser uses ultrasonic vibrations to turn water and essential oils into a fine mist that is released into the air. To diffuse oils, mix a few drops of oil with water that is set to a certain level in the diffuser to disperse oil particles in the air for you to breathe in. Aromatherapy diffusers come in different shapes and sizes and can be time controlled with a remote

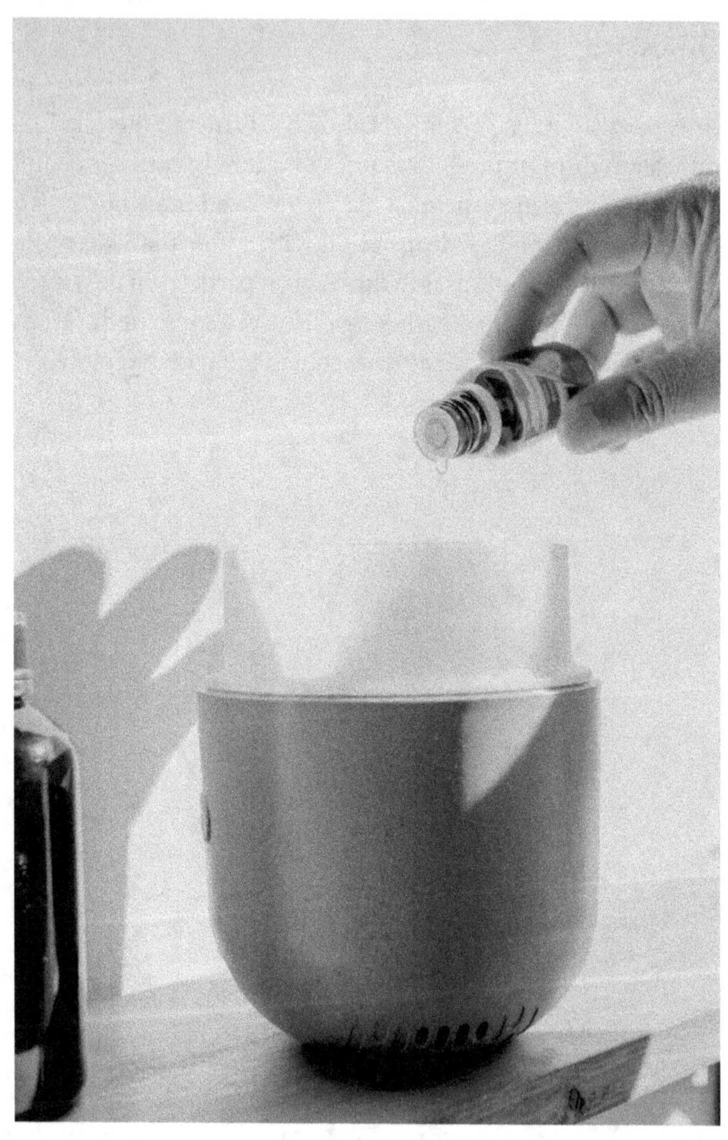

Inhalatio

:

The therapeutic benefits of essential oils can be enjoyed by inhaling them. You can open the top of the essential oil bottle and take a few deep breaths of the oil. Another option is steam inhalation, where you add a few drops of oil to a bowl of hot water, cover your head with a towel, and inhale the steam. Aromatherapy jewelry, such as bracelets and necklaces, are also designed to hold essential oils, so you can wear them and enjoy the benefits throughout the day.

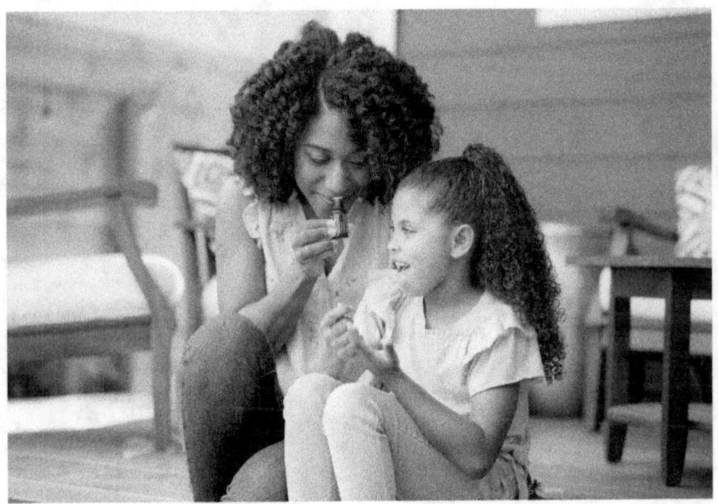

You should consult with a health care provider before using essential oils, especially if you are pregnant, nursing, or have a pre-existing medical condition. The health care provider can give specific guidance and advice on the safe and appropriate use of essential oils based on your needs

Eight

Chemical free home

Reducing toxins in your home can improve your health and well-being, but it can be overwhelming to know where to start. Every little effort can go a long way. There are many different essential oils you can incorporate into your cleaning products and also make your own products have a chemical-free home. It can offer so many health benefits in making your home safer and removing toxins from your home. [5] Here are some easy ways to incorporate essential oils into your cleaning routine and create a safer, chemical-free home.

There are many different ways to help minimize toxic items in your home. Essential oils can boost benefits in your house. Reducing toxins in your home can seem like a daunting task, but incorporating essential oils into your cleaning routine can help make your home safer and healthier. Here are some easy ways to get started.

You can add a few drops of oils in different cleaning products to help clean different rooms. Laundry rooms are a great area to start using essential oils. The fresh smell of clean clothes can always make a mom smile. The chemicals in your detergent can be harsh and cause skin irritations, so less exposure to harsh chemicals can go a long way. Applying lemongrass essential oil on wool dryer balls is also a great option to use in the dryer to eliminate the use of dryer sheets.

Creating a non-toxic disinfectant spray can help you get those counters and floors clean. Lavender and tea tree oils have natural disinfecting powers. You can make a spray with a mixture of vinegar and your choice of oil and create a disinfectant solution. Lemon oil and peppermint oils are also other options to use on countertops, bathroom use, and to clean floors. Lemon oil has multiple uses for cleaning, and it can help those stale smells and replace them with a fresh smell. You can add a few drops to any cleaner and use it around the house.

Diffuse essential oils to bring a fresh scent to your home. Freshening the air in your home is very important, and it brings a clean atmosphere when you walk into your home and breath in a great smell. Diffusing oils is a great way to freshen up a room. Lemon, lemongrass, vanilla, lavender, peppermint, and orange oils are great choices of oils to mix or use alone.

For more information on the benefits of using essential oils and cleaning, check out reputable sources such as the Environmental Working Group (EWG) or the National Association for Holistic Aromatherapy.

Nine

DIY Essential Oil recipe

Mothers strive for a safe and comfortable living space that promotes physical and emotional wellness for themselves and their loved ones. The use of essential oils is one of the most natural ways to have non-toxic health and safe intake in your home. Below are a few recipes for getting the best rest, cleanliness, health, and happiness for the family.

DIY recipes

Essential oils can be mixed to make the perfect recipe to target specific needs of what areas you want to improve in your life. Below are some mixes that add a little extra natural scent to your home.

Bedtime Sleepy Spray: glass spray bottle + 20 drops of lavender, cedarwood, tangerine, roman/german chamomile

Happiness: Lavender + Bergamot Oil

Mama belly rub can be a wonderful recipe, especially after pregnancy [17]

Recipe: Glass bottle + ½ cup of cocoa butter, ½ cup of shea butter, ¼ cup olive oil, 1 tbsp Vitamin E, 3-5 drops geranium oil, 3-5 droves lavender oil

- "Bathroom bomb" peppermint+lavender + eucalyptus+ lemongrass
- "Stinky shoes" lemon+ eucalyptus clove+cinnamon + rosemary
- "Bug be gone."
- "Heavenly hair" Rosemary oil+ Lavender oil+ Ylang Ylang oil + add Castor oil and mix in a glass bottle

Kid DIY fun essential oil ideas

There are many fund DIY essential oil ideas that kids can participate in to make and enjoy as arts and crafts.

1. Scented play dough: Make your own playdough and add a few drops of your favorite essential oil for a sensory experience.

2. Bath bombs: combine baking soda, citric acid, and your favorite essential oil to make a bath bomb. Kids will enjoy watching the bath bomb fizz and love the scents during bath time.
3. Monster spray can be a creative way to help kids overcome their fears of monsters in the closet or under the bed. Lavender Monster Spray: add ten drops of lavender oil to a spray bottle filled with water.

Celebrities Essential Oils Hacks

Essential oils are very popular nowadays. They are in many products that we use daily. It is no surprise that along with the modern moms' love of oils, celebrities have dabbled into the sweet scents of aromatherapy and essential oils. [15] Here are a few celebrities who enjoy essential oils and have shared some hacks on how they use them daily.

- Daphne Oz reveals using lavender oil for healing kitchen burns. She also puts a few drops of lavender oil in her vacuum bag to have a pleasant non-toxic aroma in her home.

- Katie Couric also loves lavender oil and uses it in her bath products.

- Kerry Washington uses a few essential oil blends, such as Joy Oil, on her nightstand. She uses oils topically and diffuses oils.

- Ellen Pompeo uses a few drops of sage oil, water, and soap when she cleans her floors, and she enjoys the scent it brings to her home.

- Robin Roberts diffuses lavender oil, and it helps her have a good night's sleep.

- Victoria Beckham talks about beauty products with essential oils such as cypress and citrus oils that boost skin appearance.

- Jenna Dewan enjoys thieves oil as an immune booster. She uses lavender oil in her bath, and rose oil also greatly affects mood. She also enjoys wearing lemon and grapefruit oils and likes the citrus scent

Eleven

Essential Oil dictionary A–Z. Here are some common oils that are great to have in your oil cabinet to reach in those most needed moments

A - Angelica- relieves stress and anxiety

B- Basil- energizes, repels insects, eliminators, odors, soothes headaches
Bergamot- reduces inflammation, promotes positive mood, skin support, helps sore throats
Blue Tansy- antihistamine, skin support

C- Cardamom- supports digestion; lower blood pressure
Cinnamon Bark- assists with stress, respiratory health-

clear airways
   Copaiba- pain relief, strep throat, heals wounds, anti-inflammatory

D- Dill- helps with skin appearance; can be added to soups

E- Eucalyptus Radiata- joint and muscle pain, relieves headache, cold and cough support

F- Frankincense- skin support, respiratory care, reduces stress

G- German Chamomile- indigestion, nausea, skin support for eczema or rashes
   Ginger- treats upset stomach; respiratory care, heart health, anxiety relief

H- Helichrysum- beauty and skin support, pain reducing, wound healing, anti-inflammatory
   Hyssop- aging support, muscle spasms, cramps, arthritis

I- Idaho Blue Spruce- relieves tension, relaxation and peacefulness

J- Jasmine- skin health, assists with low energy levels, sleep support, hormone support

L- Lavender- promotes relaxation, sleep support, allergies, skin healing
   Lemon- antibacterial, skin support, helps nausea, sore throats

Lemongrass- relieve stress, assists with digestive problems

M- Manuka- antiseptic, skin support, antibacterial
Marjoram- digestive support (indigestion, constipation), heals fungal infections
Myrrh- heals skin, helps pain and swelling, kills bacteria, parasites
N- Nutmeg- lower blood pressure, oral care support
O- Orange- uplifts mood, skin support, used in house cleaners, stomach ache support
Oregano- antiviral; fights bacteria – "hot oil"

P- Palo Santo- treats colds, flu, headaches, asthma, mental health support
Peppermint- treats headache, muscle and joint pain, pain reducer, digestion support

R- Roman Chamomile- soothes muscles, reduces inflammation
Rose- beauty and skin support, relieves spasms, reduces inflammation
Rosemary- pain reliever, hair growth, stress relief, reduces inflammation

S- Sacred Frankincense- immune system support, aging support
Sage- muscle and joint pain support, skin healing, eliminates toxins

T- Tangerine- Wound hearing, skin support, antifungal

Thyme- antifungal, antibacterial

V- Vanilla- helps muscle tension, stress relief, lowers blood pressure
    Vetiver- stress relief, support for sleep, joint and muscle pain

W- Wintergreen- skin support, headache, colic, sore throat, bacterial infection

Y- Ylang Ylang- insect repellant, mental health support, lowers blood pressure

Twelve

Conclusion

Essential oils can be a natural and effective way for mothers to utilize the best natural way to promote their well-being and family. The purpose of this book is to give guidance on the many different benefits and areas of life where essential oils can be applied. You can explore a wide range of topics, from the history of essential oils and the top essential oils for immunity, sleep, mental health, beauty, digestion, men's health, DIY recipes, and much more. This book is a valuable tool for mothers looking to find all-natural ways to enhance their physical and emotional well-being and their children, spouses, and loved ones.

It is also important to note that essential oils should always be used safely and responsibly. The FDA does not regulate essential oils. If a mom is considering using essential oils, it is critical to seek advice from a qualified healthcare provider and to follow proper usage guidelines. Pregnant and breastfeeding women should be cautious and seek medical advice before using essential oils. When following safety guidelines for using essential oils safely, moms can use them confidently in their daily family life routines and enjoy the many benefits essential oils offer. It is also important to choose high-quality oils when selecting the right oil option. Look for high-quality oils that are 100% pure and therapeutic grade, as these are the safest and most effective oils to use.

I hope this book will serve as a valuable resource for moms and their family members looking to improve their overall health and wellness naturally and healthily. By utilizing the power and strength of essential oils, mothers can take control of their well-being and enjoy the many benefits essential oils offer for a happier, healthier life. By following the guidelines, tips, knowledge, and recommendations presented in this book, mothers can be confident to incorporate essential oils into their daily routines and use them safely and effectively to see the long-term natural effects they can have for themselves and their loved ones. It takes some patience and practice, but with time and willingness to learn, you can discover the many benefits of essential oils for a healthy and happier life. Wouldn't you prefer a natural and healthy method to prevent illness, alleviate pain, and give you a more relaxing and calm way to live? Then indulge in the natural and aromatic world of essential oils to pamper yourself and your loved ones.

If you enjoyed this book and it was useful to you, I would appreciate it if you wrote a favorable review on Amazon.

Thirteen

References

1. Essential oil. (2023). Merriam Webster. Retrieved March 30, 2023, from https://www.merriam-webster.com/dictionary/essential%20oil

2. Loving essential oils. (2023). Loving Essential Oils. Retrieved March 30, 2023, from https://www.lovingessentialoils.com

3. 10 DIY essential oil crafts. (2021, May 18). Hearth & Vine. Retrieved March 30, 2023, from https://hearthandvine.com/top-10-projects-using-essential-oils/

4.History of essential oils. (2023). Essential Oils Academy. Retrieved March 30, 2023, from https://essentialoilsacademy.com/history

5. Why every mom needs try essential oils. (2023). The Military Wife. Retrieved March 30, 2023, from https://the militarywifeandmom.com/best-essential-oil-uses-mom s/

6.11 Essential Oils: Their benefits and how to use them. (2021, December 14). Cleveland Clinic. Retrieved March 30, 2023, from https://health.clevelandclinic.org/essenti al-oils-101-do-they-work-how-do-you-use-them/

7.Health benefits of essential oils. (2022, November 28). Nourish by WebMD. Retrieved March 30, 2023, from https://www.webmd.com/diet/health-benefits-essentia l-oils#:~:text=Essential%20oils%20smell%20great%2C%2 0reduce,many%20medicinal%20and%20recreational%20 uses

8. https://www.healthline.com/health/cold-flu/essentia l-oils-for-colds#benefits
   Can essential oils treat or prevent colds. (2023). Health-line. Retrieved March 30, 2023, from https://www.healt hline.com/health/cold-flu/essential-oils-for-colds#bene fits

9.The 7 best essential oils for men. (2022, June 15). Radha Beauty. Retrieved March 30, 2023, from https://www.r adhabeauty.com/blogs/radha-blog/the-7-best-essential- oils-for-men

10. Riddle, J. (2022, September 8). Essential Oils for Children's Sleep — Mālama Momma. Mālama Momma. Retrieved March 30, 2023, from https://www.malamamo mma.com/blog/essential-oils-to-help-children-sleep

11. Best 8 essential oils for cuts and wounds. (2020, November 23). Aromas. Retrieved April 1, 2023, from https://aromis.co/blog/best-8-essential-oils-for-cuts-an d-wounds/

12. Are essential oils safe? 13 things to know before use. (2019, April 26). Healthline. Retrieved April 1, 2023, from https://www.healthline.com/health/are-essential-oils-safe#topical-use

13. 7 must know revitalizing essential oils good for skin. (2021, September 17). Fresh Mommy Blog. Retrieved April 2, 2023, from https://freshmommyblog.com/7-must-kno w-revitalizing-essential-oils-good-for-skin/

14. Aromatherapy. (n.d.). The Wholistic Esthetician. Retrieved April 2, 2023, from https://thewholisticesthe tician.com/aromatherapy

15. 7 Celebrities who love essential oils more than you do. (2019, September 26). First for Women. Retrieved April 2, 2023, from https://www.firstforwomen.com/gallery/en tertainment/celebrities-who-use-essential-oils-172818

16. https://www.healthline.com/health/are-essential-oi

ls-safe#infants-and-children

17. 15 DIY Essential Oil Recipes for gifts and holidays. (2019, May 24). Mama Natural. Retrieved April 2, 2023, from https://www.mamanatural.com/diy-essential-oil-recipes/